APA Mastery Manual 7th edition 2024

Strategies, Examples, and Best Practices for Successful Scholarly Writing

Introduction

- Brief overview of the APA Manual 7th edition

- Importance of adhering to APA style guidelines

- Purpose of the guide

Chapter 1: Basics of APA Style

- Overview of APA style

- General formatting guidelines

- Title page, abstract, body text, and references

- In-text citations

Chapter 2: Manuscript Structure and Content

- Title page formatting

- Abstract formatting and content

- Body text structure (headings, subheadings, paragraphs)

- Tables and figures

- Appendices

Chapter 3: In-Text Citations

- Overview of in-text citations

- Author-date citation system

- Rules for citing different types of sources (books, journal articles, websites, etc.)

- Examples of in-text citations

Chapter 4: Reference List

- Overview of reference list formatting

- Rules for listing different types of sources (books, journal articles, websites, etc.)

- Examples of reference list entries

Chapter 5: Writing Style and Grammar

- Clarity and conciseness in writing

- Grammar and punctuation guidelines

- Avoiding bias in language

- Writing style tips

Chapter 6: Ethical and Legal Considerations

- Plagiarism and self-plagiarism

- Ethical considerations in research and writing

- Copyright and fair use guidelines

Chapter 7: Common Errors and FAQs

- Common mistakes in APA formatting

- Frequently asked questions about APA style

- Troubleshooting tips

Appendix: Sample Papers

- Sample APA-formatted paper

- Examples of different elements such as title page, abstract, citations, and reference list

Glossary

- Definitions of key terms and concepts used in the APA Manual

References

- List of sources consulted in creating the guide

INTRODUCTION

Welcome to the "APA Mastery Manual 7th edition 2024." This comprehensive guide aims to provide clear and concise instructions on adhering to the guidelines outlined in the American Psychological Association (APA) Manual, 7th edition. Whether you're a student, researcher, or academic writer, mastering APA style is essential for effectively communicating your ideas and ensuring the credibility of your work.

Purpose of the Guide

The purpose of this guide is to demystify the complexities of APA style and empower you to confidently apply its principles in your writing. By breaking down the key components of APA formatting, citation, and writing style, this guide aims to equip you with the knowledge and skills necessary to produce well-structured, academically rigorous papers.

Importance of APA Style

Adhering to APA style guidelines is crucial for several reasons. First and foremost, it promotes clarity and consistency in scholarly communication, allowing readers to easily locate and understand the information presented in your work. Additionally, following APA style helps to maintain academic integrity by providing proper credit to the sources you've consulted and avoiding plagiarism.

Whether you're formatting a research paper, crafting an annotated bibliography, or preparing a manuscript for publication, understanding APA style is indispensable. This guide will serve as your roadmap to navigating the intricacies of APA formatting, citation, and writing conventions, enabling you to produce polished and professional academic documents.

Let's embark on this journey to master the nuances of APA style and elevate the quality of your scholarly writing.

CHAPTER 1: BASICS OF APA STYLE

In this chapter, we will delve into the fundamental principles of APA style, covering general formatting guidelines, title page requirements, and the structure of an APA-formatted paper. Understanding these basics is essential for ensuring consistency and professionalism in your academic writing.

Overview of APA Style

APA style, developed by the American Psychological Association, is a set of guidelines for formatting academic papers and citing sources in the social sciences. It provides standards for writing and organizing research papers, manuscripts, essays, and other scholarly documents.

General Formatting Guidelines

APA style specifies various formatting conventions to create uniformity and enhance readability in academic writing. These guidelines include:

- Margins: Use 1-inch margins on all sides of the paper.

- Font: Use a clear and legible font such as Times New Roman or Arial, size 12.

- Spacing: Double-space the entire paper, including the title page, abstract, main text, references, and appendices.

- Alignment: Align text to the left margin; do not justify the text.

- Page Numbers: Include page numbers in the upper right corner of each page, starting with the title page.

Title Page

The title page is the first page of an APA-formatted paper and serves as the cover page. It includes essential information such as the title of the paper, author's name, institutional affiliation (if applicable), and author note (if necessary).

Title Page Elements:

- Title: Concisely summarize the main idea of your paper.

- Author's Name: Include the author's full name.

- Institutional Affiliation: Indicate the author's institutional affiliation (e.g., university or organization).

- Author Note: Provide additional information about the author(s), such as departmental affiliation, contact information, or acknowledgments (optional).

Structure of an APA-formatted Paper

An APA-formatted paper typically consists of the following sections:

1. Title Page

2. Abstract

3. Body Text

4. References

Each section serves a specific purpose and follows prescribed formatting guidelines. Understanding the structure of an APA paper is essential for organizing your thoughts and presenting your research effectively.

In the following chapters, we will explore each section in detail, providing step-by-step instructions and examples to help you master the nuances of APA style.

CHAPTER 2: MANUSCRIPT STRUCTURE AND CONTENT

In this chapter, we will discuss the structure and content of an APA-formatted manuscript. From the title page to the appendices, each component plays a crucial role in presenting your research effectively and adhering to APA style guidelines.

Title Page Formatting

The title page is the first page of your manuscript and serves as the cover page. It includes essential information such as the title of the paper, author's name, institutional affiliation (if applicable), and author note (if necessary).

Title Page Elements:

- Title: Concisely summarize the main idea of your paper.

- Author's Name: Include the author's full name.

- Institutional Affiliation: Indicate the author's institutional affiliation (e.g., university or organization).

- Author Note: Provide additional information about the author(s), such as departmental affiliation, contact information, or acknowledgments (optional).

Abstract Formatting and Content

The abstract is a concise summary of your paper, providing an overview of the research question, methods, results, and conclusions. It should be written in a clear, concise, and informative manner, typically containing 150-250 words.

Abstract Elements:

- Background: Briefly introduce the topic and research question.

- Methods: Describe the research design, participants, measures, and procedures.

- Results: Summarize the key findings of the study.

- Conclusions: Discuss the implications of the findings and future directions.

Body Text Structure

The body of your paper should be organized into sections and subsections, following a hierarchical structure. Use clear and descriptive headings to guide readers through the content and facilitate navigation.

Body Text Elements:

- Introduction: Provide background information, state the research question or hypothesis, and outline the purpose of the study.

- Methods: Describe the research design, participants, measures, and procedures in detail.

- Results: Present the findings of the study, including statistical analyses and data summaries.

- Discussion: Interpret the results, discuss their implications, and relate them to previous research.

- Conclusion: Summarize the main findings and highlight their significance.

Tables and Figures

Tables and figures are used to present numerical data, complex information, or visual representations of results. They should be numbered consecutively and accompanied by clear and concise captions that explain their content.

Table and Figure Elements:

- Table: Organize data in rows and columns for easy comparison and reference.

- Figure: Use graphs, charts, or images to visually represent data or concepts.

Appendices

Appendices contain supplementary materials that are not essential to the main text but provide additional context or information. Common appendix content includes raw data, survey instruments, and detailed methodological descriptions.

Appendix Elements:

- Appendix Title: Clearly label each appendix with a descriptive title.

- Content: Include supplementary materials such as tables, figures, or additional analyses.

Understanding the structure and content of an APA-formatted manuscript is essential for organizing your research effectively and presenting it in a clear and professional manner.

In the following chapters, we will delve deeper into specific elements of manuscript preparation, providing detailed guidelines and examples to help you navigate the complexities of APA style.

CHAPTER 3: IN-TEXT CITATIONS

Overview of In-Text Citations

In-text citations serve multiple purposes in academic writing. They not only attribute credit to the original sources of information but also provide readers with a roadmap to locate the full bibliographic details in the reference list. In APA style, in-text citations generally consist of the author's last name and the publication year of the source, both enclosed in parentheses, e.g., (Smith, 2019). However, the format of the in-text citation may vary depending on factors such as the type of source, the number of authors, and whether direct quotations or paraphrased information is being cited.

In-text citations are crucial for maintaining academic integrity and avoiding plagiarism. By clearly indicating when you are drawing upon someone else's ideas or research, you demonstrate ethical scholarship and contribute to the credibility of your own work. Therefore, understanding the nuances of APA in-text citation guidelines is essential for scholars, researchers, and students alike. This chapter will explore the various aspects of in-text citations in detail, providing guidelines and examples to help you navigate this important aspect of academic writing effectively.

Examples of In-Text Citations

In-text citations in APA style can take various forms depending on the structure of the source being cited. Here are examples of different cases:

1. Single Author:

   - Example: (Smith, 2019)

2. Two Authors:

   - Example: (Johnson & Lee, 2020)

3. Three or More Authors (First Citation):

   - Example: (Brown et al., 2018)

4. Three or More Authors (Subsequent Citations):

   - Example: (Brown et al., 2018)

5. Organization as Author:

   - Example: (American Psychological Association [APA], 2020)

6. No Author:

   - Example: ("Title of Article," 2021)

7. Multiple Works by the Same Author(s):

   - Example: (Smith, 2019a; Smith, 2019b)

8. Direct Quotations:

   - Example: (Johnson & Lee, 2020, p. 25)

9. Works with Specific Parts (e.g., Chapters, Sections):

   - Example: (Brown, 2018, Chapter 3)

10. Personal Communication:

   - Example: (J. Doe, personal communication, May 5, 2024)

These examples cover a range of scenarios encountered when citing sources in APA style. Understanding how to format in-text citations correctly ensures that your writing is clear, accurate, and compliant with APA guidelines.

Guidelines for In-Text Citations

In addition to understanding the various formats of in-text citations, it's essential to follow specific guidelines for integrating citations smoothly into your text. Here are some key guidelines to keep in mind:

1. Place Citations Immediately After the Information Being Cited: In-text citations should appear immediately after the information being cited, usually at the end of the sentence or clause.

2. Use Parentheses for Citations: Enclose in-text citations in parentheses, including the author's last name and the publication year. Separate multiple citations with semicolons.

3. Include Page Numbers for Direct Quotations: When citing direct quotations, include the page number(s) in the in-text citation after the publication year, separated by a comma.

4. Integrate Citations Seamlessly into the Text: Avoid interrupting the flow of your writing with overly frequent or awkwardly placed citations. Instead, integrate citations seamlessly into your sentences, using signal phrases to introduce them when necessary.

5. Provide Enough Information for Readers to Locate the Source: Ensure that your in-text citations provide enough information for readers to locate the corresponding entry in the reference list. Include the author's last name and the publication year, as well as specific page numbers for direct quotations.

6. Be Consistent in Citation Style: Maintain consistency in your citation style throughout your paper. Use the same format for in-text citations within the same paper and follow APA guidelines for citing different types of sources.

7. Use Abbreviations for Group Authors: When citing group authors, such as organizations or government agencies, use abbreviations or acronyms in subsequent citations if they are lengthy or frequently cited.

By following these guidelines, you can ensure that your in-text citations are accurate, clear, and properly integrated into your writing, enhancing the credibility and professionalism of your work. Understanding the nuances of in-text citation formatting is essential for effective scholarly communication in APA style.

Incorporating In-Text Citations into Your Writing

Now that we've explored the various formats and guidelines for in-text citations, let's discuss strategies for effectively incorporating them into your writing:

1. Introduce Sources with Signal Phrases: Signal phrases are introductory phrases or clauses that provide context for the citation. They help smoothly integrate the citation into your sentence and indicate to the reader that you are referencing an external source. Examples of signal phrases include "According to," "As Smith (2019) argues," or "In a recent study by Johnson and Lee (2020),..."

2. Provide Context for Each Citation: After introducing a source with a signal phrase, briefly summarize the key point or findings of the source before or after the citation. This ensures that readers understand why the source is relevant to your argument and how it contributes to your overall discussion.

3. Use In-Text Citations Sparingly: While it's essential to support your arguments with evidence from credible sources, avoid overloading your writing with excessive citations. Instead, focus on incorporating citations strategically to reinforce key points or provide evidence for contentious claims.

4. Blend Quotations and Paraphrases: In addition to direct quotations, incorporate paraphrases and summaries of source material into your writing. Paraphrasing allows you to convey the ideas of other authors in your own words while still acknowledging the source with an in-text citation.

5. Maintain a Consistent Citation Style: Ensure that your in-text citations follow a consistent format throughout your paper. Consistency in citation style enhances the readability of your writing and demonstrates attention to detail.

6. Check for Accuracy and Completeness: Before finalizing your paper, review your in-text citations to ensure that they are accurate and complete. Verify that you have included the author's last name, publication year, and page number (if applicable) for each citation, and cross-reference them with the corresponding entries in your reference list.

By incorporating these strategies into your writing process, you can effectively integrate in-text citations into your paper, support your arguments with evidence from credible sources, and enhance the clarity and credibility of your work. In-text citations not only demonstrate your engagement with existing literature but also contribute to the academic integrity of your writing.

Avoiding Plagiarism with In-Text Citations

In-text citations play a crucial role in academic writing by attributing credit to the original sources of information and ideas. However, they also serve another important purpose: preventing plagiarism. Plagiarism occurs when you use someone else's words or ideas without proper attribution, and it can have serious consequences for your academic and professional reputation.

Here are some key ways in which in-text citations help you avoid plagiarism:

1. Giving Credit to the Original Author: By including in-text citations whenever you use someone else's words, ideas, or findings, you give credit to the original author or source. This demonstrates academic integrity and honesty in your writing.

2. Differentiating Your Ideas from Others': In-text citations help distinguish your original ideas and contributions from those of other authors. They provide a clear trail for readers to follow, showing where your ideas end and the cited sources begin.

3. Providing Evidence for Your Claims: In-text citations lend credibility to your arguments by providing evidence from credible sources to support your claims. They show that your ideas are grounded in existing research and scholarship.

4. Avoiding Accidental Plagiarism: Even if you don't intend to plagiarize, it's possible to accidentally use someone else's words or ideas without proper attribution. In-text citations act as a safeguard against accidental plagiarism by ensuring that you acknowledge the sources of information you've used in your writing.

5. Respecting Intellectual Property Rights: Properly citing your sources demonstrates respect for the intellectual property rights of other authors and researchers. It acknowledges their contributions to the scholarly conversation and honors the principles of academic honesty and integrity.

In summary, in-text citations are not only a requirement of academic writing but also a fundamental tool for avoiding plagiarism and upholding ethical standards. By incorporating in-text citations into your writing effectively and consistently, you demonstrate your commitment to academic integrity and contribute to the integrity of the scholarly community as a whole.

Understanding and Avoiding Common Errors

While in-text citations are essential for maintaining academic integrity and avoiding plagiarism, there are several common errors that writers may encounter. Being aware of these errors can help you avoid them in your own writing. Here are some common mistakes to watch out for:

1. Missing or Incomplete Citations: Forgetting to include in-text citations or omitting essential information such as the author's last name or publication year can lead to incomplete or inaccurate citations. Always double-check your citations to ensure that they are complete and accurate.

2. Incorrect Formatting: In-text citations must be formatted correctly according to APA style guidelines. This includes placing the citation within parentheses, using the appropriate punctuation, and following the prescribed format for different types of sources. Refer to the APA Manual or a reliable style guide for guidance on proper citation formatting.

3. Overreliance on Direct Quotations: While direct quotations can be useful for capturing the precise wording of an author's argument, overusing them can detract from your own voice and analysis. Aim to incorporate paraphrases and summaries of source material into your writing, using direct quotations sparingly and selectively.

4. Failure to Integrate Citations Seamlessly: In-text citations should be seamlessly integrated into your writing, rather than inserted awkwardly or disruptively. Use signal phrases, transitions, and sentence structure to smoothly incorporate citations into your text, avoiding abrupt shifts or interruptions in your writing flow.

5. Inconsistent Citation Style: Consistency is key when it comes to citation style. Ensure that your in-text citations follow a consistent format throughout your paper, including consistent use of author names, publication years, and punctuation. Inconsistencies in citation style can confuse readers and detract from the professionalism of your writing.

6. Misuse of Secondary Sources: When citing sources, it's important to distinguish between primary and secondary sources. Avoid citing secondary sources (i.e., sources that cite other sources) unless absolutely necessary. Whenever possible, go directly to the original source to verify the information and provide a more reliable citation.

By being mindful of these common errors and taking steps to avoid them, you can ensure that your in-text citations are accurate, clear, and properly integrated into your writing. Remember that in-text citations are not only a requirement of academic writing but also a reflection of your commitment to ethical scholarship and academic integrity.

Reviewing In-Text Citations: Frequently Asked Questions

As you navigate the complexities of in-text citations in APA style, you may encounter various questions and uncertainties. Here are some frequently asked questions (FAQs) to help clarify common issues:

1. When should I use an in-text citation?

  - In-text citations should be used whenever you directly quote, paraphrase, or summarize information from a source. Essentially, any time you use someone else's ideas, words, or findings in your writing, you need to provide an in-text citation to credit the original author.

2. Do I need to include page numbers in every in-text citation?

  - Page numbers are typically included in in-text citations for direct quotations. However, they may not be necessary for paraphrases or summaries, especially if the information is from a source without page numbers (e.g., a website). Follow APA guidelines and provide page numbers when available and relevant.

3. What should I do if the source has multiple authors?

- If a source has two authors, include both authors' last names in the in-text citation, joined by an ampersand (&). For sources with three or more authors, use the first author's last name followed by "et al." in subsequent citations.

4. How do I cite sources with no author or date?

- If a source has no author, use the title of the work in the in-text citation. If the source has no date, use "n.d." (for "no date") in place of the publication year. For example, ("Title of Article," n.d.).

5. What should I do if I'm citing a source that cites another source?

- Whenever possible, try to locate and cite the original source directly. If you cannot access the original source, you can cite the secondary source in your text and include both the original and secondary sources in your reference list. Follow APA guidelines for citing secondary sources.

6. How do I cite personal communications in-text?

- Personal communications, such as interviews, emails, or conversations, should be cited in-text with the name of the person and the date of the communication. Include a note specifying the nature of the communication (e.g., "personal communication," "email," "interview").

By familiarizing yourself with these FAQs and consulting reputable APA style resources when needed, you can confidently navigate the intricacies of in-text citations and ensure that your writing adheres to APA guidelines with accuracy and clarity.

Here are more frequently asked questions (FAQs) regarding in-text citations in APA style:

7. How do I cite a source with multiple works by the same author?

- When citing multiple works by the same author, differentiate them by adding lowercase letters (a, b, c, etc.) after the publication year. Order the citations alphabetically by title if the same author has multiple works published in the same year.

8. Should I include in-text citations in the abstract?

- In general, in-text citations are not included in the abstract. However, if the abstract contains specific information that is directly quoted or paraphrased from a source, it should be cited following APA guidelines.

9. Can I cite sources in the reference list that are not cited in-text?

- It is generally recommended to only include sources in the reference list that are cited in-text. However, if you have consulted additional sources that have informed your understanding of the topic but are not directly cited in your paper, you may include them in a separate section titled "Additional Reading" or "Further Reading" instead of the reference list.

10. What should I do if I'm unsure how to cite a specific type of source?

- If you encounter a source type or citation scenario that you're unsure how to handle, consult the APA Manual or reputable APA style guides for guidance. You can also seek assistance from academic librarians, writing centers, or online resources dedicated to APA style.

11. How do I cite sources in a non-English language?

- When citing sources in a non-English language, provide the original title in the in-text citation followed by an English translation in square brackets if necessary. Ensure that the citation includes all the necessary information required by APA style guidelines.

12. Can I use et al. in the reference list?

  - While "et al." is commonly used in in-text citations for sources with three or more authors, it should not be used in the reference list. List all authors' names in the reference list up to 20 authors. If a work has more than 20 authors, list the first 19 authors followed by an ellipsis (...) and then the last author's name.

By addressing these frequently asked questions, you can enhance your understanding of in-text citations in APA style and effectively apply them in your academic writing with confidence and accuracy. Continuously referring to APA style resources and seeking clarification when needed will help you navigate the complexities of citation formatting successfully.

CHAPTER 4: REFERENCE LIST

In this chapter, we will delve into the intricacies of creating a reference list in APA style. The reference list is a critical component of academic writing as it provides readers with the necessary information to locate and verify the sources cited in your paper. Properly formatting your reference list is essential for ensuring accuracy, consistency, and adherence to APA guidelines. This chapter will cover everything you need to know about formatting your reference list, including the essential elements of each reference entry and specific formatting rules for different types of sources.

Elements of a Reference Entry

1. Author(s):

   - For books, articles, and other written works authored by individuals, include the author's last name followed by initials (e.g., Smith, J. R.). Use an ampersand (&) instead of "and" when citing multiple authors within parentheses.

   - For group authors or organizations, use the full name of the group or organization as the author. If the group author has a well-known abbreviation or acronym, you can use it in subsequent citations.

2. Publication Year:

   - The publication year indicates when the source was published or released. It follows the author's name and is enclosed in parentheses. If multiple works by the same author are cited, list them in chronological order, with the earliest publication year first.

3. Title:

   - The title of the source should be provided in sentence case, where only the first word of the title and proper nouns are capitalized. It is italicized for books, journals, and other standalone works.

   - For articles, chapters, or other shorter works published within larger works, such as journals or edited books, the title is not italicized but enclosed in quotation marks.

4. Source Information:

- Depending on the type of source, additional information may be included in the reference entry to help readers identify and locate the source.

- For books, include the book title (if different from the main title), edition (if not the first edition), and publisher. The publisher's name is usually abbreviated and followed by a colon.

- For articles, include the journal title (italicized), volume and issue numbers (in parentheses), and page range (inclusive page numbers). Use the abbreviation "pp." for page numbers.

5. DOI or URL (if applicable):

- For online sources that have a DOI (Digital Object Identifier), include it in the reference entry. The DOI provides a permanent link to the source and helps ensure its accessibility over time.

- If a DOI is not available, include the URL (web address) of the source. Ensure that the URL is formatted correctly and leads directly to the source. Avoid including unnecessary characters or tracking information in the URL.

6. Access Date (if applicable):

- If the source is retrieved from a website or online database where the content may change over time, include the date you accessed the source. This helps provide context for the reader and indicates the version of the source you consulted.

7. Location Information (if applicable):

- For sources such as books, reports, or theses that have a physical location, such as a city or state, include this information in the reference entry. This helps readers identify where the source was published or produced.

- The location information typically follows the publisher's name and is separated by a colon. For example, "New York, NY: Publisher Name."

8. Edition (if applicable):

- If the source is a subsequent edition of a book, include the edition number after the title of the book. Abbreviate "edition" to "ed." and place it in parentheses after the title.

  - For example, "Title of Book (2nd ed.)."

9. Volume and Issue Numbers (for Journal Articles):

  - When citing journal articles, include the volume and issue numbers of the journal where the article was published. The volume number is typically followed by the issue number in parentheses.

  - For example, "Journal Title, 10(3), 100-120."

10. Page Range (for Articles):

  - Provide the inclusive page numbers of the article within the journal or other periodical. The page range indicates the specific pages where the article appears.

  - Use "pp." before the page numbers to indicate multiple pages. For example, "pp. 100-120."

11. Publisher's Name (for Books):

  - Include the publisher's name after the title of the book. The publisher's name is usually abbreviated and followed by a colon.

  - For example, "Publisher Name."

12. DOI (Digital Object Identifier):

  - The DOI is a unique alphanumeric string assigned to digital documents to provide a persistent link to the source. Include the DOI if available, as it provides a reliable means for readers to access the source online.

  - The DOI is typically included at the end of the reference entry, preceded by "doi:" For example, "doi:10.1111/j.1467-8535.2012.01354.x."

Formatting Reference Entries for Different Source Types

In this section, we will explore the specific formatting guidelines for creating reference entries for various types of sources commonly cited in academic writing. Each source type has unique formatting requirements, and understanding how to format reference entries correctly ensures consistency and accuracy in your reference list. We will cover the formatting guidelines for books, journal articles, webpages, reports, and other common source types.

Books

When formatting reference entries for books in APA style, follow these guidelines:

1. Format for Single Author:

   - Author(s): Author's Last Name, Initial(s).

   - Publication Year: (Year).

   - Title: Title of Book (Italicized).

   - Edition (if applicable): (Edition).

   - Location: Publisher.

   Example:

   Smith, J. R. (2019). *The Art of Academic Writing* (2nd ed.). New York, NY: Academic Press.

2. Format for Two Authors:

   - Author(s): Author 1's Last Name, Initial(s), & Author 2's Last Name, Initial(s).

   - Publication Year: (Year).

   - Title: Title of Book (Italicized).

- Edition (if applicable): (Edition).

- Location: Publisher.

Example:

Johnson, A., & Lee, K. (2020). *Research Methods: A Practical Guide* (3rd ed.). Boston, MA: Research Press.

3. Format for Three or More Authors (First Citation):

- Author(s): First Author's Last Name, Initial(s), Second Author's Last Name, Initial(s), ..., & Last Author's Last Name, Initial(s).

- Publication Year: (Year).

- Title: Title of Book (Italicized).

- Edition (if applicable): (Edition).

- Location: Publisher.

Example:

Brown, P., Wilson, L., Garcia, M., & Smith, D. (2018). Social Psychology: An Introduction (6th ed.). London, UK: Pearson.

4. Format for Three or More Authors (Subsequent Citations):

- Use "et al." after the first author's name.

Example:

Brown et al. (2018) conducted a comprehensive analysis...

5. Format for Edited Book:

- Editor(s): Editor(s)' Last Name, Initial(s) (Ed. or Eds.).

- Publication Year: (Year).

- Title: Title of Book (Italicized).

- Edition (if applicable): (Edition).

- Location: Publisher.

Example:

Adams, J., & Davis, L. (Eds.). (2021). *Advances in Neuroscience* (4th ed.). Chicago, IL: Springer.

Journal Articles

When formatting reference entries for journal articles in APA style, adhere to the following guidelines:

1. Format for Print Journal Article:

   - Author(s): Author's Last Name, Initial(s).

   - Publication Year: (Year).

   - Title of Article: Article Title (Sentence Case).

   - Journal Title: *Journal Title* (Italicized), Volume Number(Issue Number), Page Range.

Example:

Smith, J. R. (2018). The impact of technology on education. *Educational Psychology Review*, 25(3), 345-360.

2. Format for Online Journal Article with DOI:

   - Author(s): Author's Last Name, Initial(s).

   - Publication Year: (Year).

   - Title of Article: Article Title (Sentence Case).

- Journal Title: *Journal Title* (Italicized), Volume Number(Issue Number), Page Range.

- DOI: doi:xxxxxxxxxx

Example:

Johnson, A., & Lee, K. (2020). Understanding student engagement in online learning. *Journal of Educational Technology*, 12(4), 112-125. doi:10.1234/jet.2020.0123

3. Format for Online Journal Article without DOI:

- Author(s): Author's Last Name, Initial(s).

- Publication Year: (Year).

- Title of Article: Article Title (Sentence Case).

- Journal Title: *Journal Title* (Italicized), Volume Number(Issue Number), Page Range.

- URL: URL of the journal homepage or the specific article.

Example:

Brown, P., & Garcia, M. (2019). The role of social media in academic communication. *Journal of Communication Studies*, 8(2), 78-92. Retrieved from https://www.journalofcommunicationstudies.com/article123

Webpages

When formatting reference entries for webpages in APA style, follow these guidelines:

1. Format for Webpage with Author(s):

- Author(s): Author's Last Name, Initial(s) or Full Name.

- Publication Year: (Year, if available).

- Title of Webpage: Title of Webpage (Sentence Case).

- Website Name: Name of Website (Italicized).

- URL: URL of the webpage.

Example:

Smith, J. (2020). *The Importance of Sleep for Academic Success*. Sleep Foundation. Retrieved from https://www.sleepfoundation.org/importance-sleep-academic-success

2. Format for Webpage without Author:

- Title of Webpage: Title of Webpage (Sentence Case).

- Website Name: Name of Website (Italicized).

- Publication Date (if available): (Year, Month Day).

- URL: URL of the webpage.

Example:

The Benefits of Meditation. (2021, April 15). Healthline. Retrieved from https://www.healthline.com/benefits-of-meditation

3. Format for Entire Website:

- Website Name: Name of Website (Italicized).

- Publication Date (if available): (Year, Month Day).

- URL: URL of the website.

Example:

Sleep Foundation. (2020). Retrieved from https://www.sleepfoundation.org/

Reports and Government Documents

When formatting reference entries for reports and government documents in APA style, adhere to the following guidelines:

1. Format for Report with an Author(s):

   - Author(s): Author's Last Name, Initial(s) or Full Name.

   - Publication Year: (Year).

   - Title of Report: Title of Report (Sentence Case).

   - Report Number (if available): Report Number.

   - Publisher: Publisher Name.

   Example:

   Smith, J. R. (2020). *Annual Report on Environmental Sustainability* (Report No. 12345). Environmental Protection Agency.

2. Format for Report without an Author:

   - Title of Report: Title of Report (Sentence Case).

   - Publication Year: (Year).

   - Report Number (if available): Report Number.

   - Publisher: Publisher Name.

   Example:

   Global Climate Change: An Overview (Report No. 98765). United Nations.

3. Format for Government Document (e.g., Bill, Law, or Regulation):

   - Jurisdiction: Jurisdiction (e.g., U.S., United Kingdom).

- Title of Document: Title of Document (Sentence Case).

- Publication Year: (Year).

- Document Number (if available): Document Number.

Example:

United States. (2020). *Coronavirus Aid, Relief, and Economic Security Act.*

Other Source Types

In this section, we will cover the formatting guidelines for reference entries of various other source types commonly cited in academic writing:

1. Format for Conference Proceedings:

   - Author(s): Author's Last Name, Initial(s) or Full Name.

   - Publication Year: (Year).

   - Title of Proceedings: Title of Proceedings (Sentence Case).

   - Conference Name: Name of Conference (Italicized).

   - Location: Location of Conference.

   - Publisher: Publisher Name.

Example:

Smith, J. R., & Johnson, A. (Eds.). (2019). *Proceedings of the International Conference on Education* (ICEDU 2019). New York, NY: Academic Press.

2. Format for Thesis or Dissertation:

   - Author: Author's Last Name, Initial(s) or Full Name.

- Publication Year: (Year).

- Title of Thesis or Dissertation: Title of Thesis or Dissertation (Sentence Case).

- Type of Work: [Master's thesis] or [Doctoral dissertation], University Name.

Example:

Brown, P. (2020). *Exploring the Impact of Online Learning on Student Engagement* [Master's thesis], University of California, Los Angeles.

3. Format for Personal Communication:

- Sender's Name: Sender's First Initial. Last Name (Personal communication, Date).

Example:

A. Johnson (Personal communication, April 1, 2024).

4. Format for Legal Cases (Court Decisions):

- Case Name v. Opposing Party: Case Name (Year).

- Volume Source Page: Volume Source Page (e.g., Volume Number, Source Abbreviation, Page Number).

Example:

Roe v. Wade (1973). 410 U.S. 113.

5. Format for Interviews:

- Interviewee's Name: Interviewee's First Initial. Last Name (Interview).

Example:

J. Smith (Interview).

CHAPTER 5: CITATIONS WITHIN THE TEXT

Basics of In-Text Citations

In-text citations are used to acknowledge the sources of information and ideas that you have used in your writing. They serve two main purposes: to give credit to the original authors and to enable readers to locate the corresponding entry in your reference list. Here are the basics of in-text citations in APA style:

1. Author-Date Format:

- In APA style, in-text citations typically include the author's last name and the publication year of the source.

- Place the author's last name and the publication year in parentheses, separated by a comma, at the end of the sentence containing the cited information.

- If the author's name is mentioned in the text, include only the publication year in parentheses.

Example:

- (Smith, 2020)

- According to Smith (2020), ...

2. Multiple Authors:

- For sources with multiple authors, include all authors' last names in the in-text citation, separated by commas, and use an ampersand (&) before the last author's name.

- If a source has three or more authors, include only the first author's last name followed by "et al." in subsequent citations.

Example:

- (Smith & Johnson, 2019)

- (Smith et al., 2018)

3. Page Numbers:

   - Include page numbers for direct quotations, paraphrases, and summaries.

   - Place the page number or page range after the publication year, separated by a comma.

   - Use the abbreviation "p." for a single page and "pp." for multiple pages.

   Example:

   - (Smith, 2020, p. 25)

   - (Johnson & Lee, 2019, pp. 45-46)

Handling Specific Citation Scenarios

In this section, we'll address specific citation scenarios that may arise when citing sources within the text:

1. Citing Sources with No Author:

   - If a source has no author, use the title (or a shortened version of the title) in place of the author's name in the in-text citation.

   - Enclose the title in quotation marks if it refers to an article, chapter, or webpage, and italicize it if it refers to a book or report.

   Example:

   - ("Title of Article," 2020)

   - (Title of Book, 2019)

2. Citing Electronic Sources with No Page Numbers:

- When citing sources without page numbers, such as websites or online articles, use paragraph numbers (if available) or another clear indicator of location.

- If paragraph numbers are not available, omit the page number element from the citation.

Example:

- (Smith, 2021, para. 4)

- (Johnson, 2020, Conclusion section)

3. Citing Secondary Sources:

- If you are citing a source that you found cited in another source (a secondary source), try to locate and cite the original source directly.

- If you cannot access the original source, use "as cited in" to indicate that you are citing the secondary source.

Example:

- (Smith, 2018, as cited in Johnson, 2020)

4. Citing Multiple Works within the Same Parentheses:

- When citing multiple works within the same parentheses, separate the citations with semicolons.

- List the citations alphabetically by the first author's last name.

Example:

- (Smith, 2019; Johnson & Lee, 2020; Brown et al., 2018)

Formatting Variations in In-Text Citations

In this section, we'll explore some variations in formatting in-text citations based on specific circumstances:

1. Citing a Corporate Author:

   - When the author of a source is a corporate entity or organization, use the full name of the organization as the author in the in-text citation.

   - If the organization's name is long or frequently cited, you may use an abbreviated form in subsequent citations.

   Example:

   - (American Psychological Association, 2020)

   - (APA, 2020)

2. Citing Electronic Sources with No Date:

   - If a source does not include a publication date, use "n.d." (no date) in place of the year in the in-text citation.

   - Provide as much detail as possible to help readers locate the source in the reference list.

   Example:

   - (Smith, n.d.)

3. Citing Translated Works:

   - When citing a translated work, include the original publication year along with the translation year in the in-text citation.

   - Place the original publication year in square brackets before the translator's name.

Example:

- (Freud, [1900] 2010)

4. Citing Personal Communications:

- Personal communications, such as interviews, emails, or phone conversations, are cited in the text only and are not included in the reference list.

- Provide the name of the person and the communication format, followed by the date of the communication.

Example:

- (J. Smith, personal communication, April 1, 2024)

CHAPTER 6: REFERENCE LIST

In this chapter, we'll focus on creating and formatting the reference list, which is a crucial component of academic writing in APA style. The reference list provides detailed information about all the sources cited in your paper, allowing readers to locate and verify the sources. We'll cover the formatting guidelines for creating a reference list, including the order of entries, formatting rules for different source types, and handling specific citation scenarios.

Structure and Formatting

The reference list in APA style is a separate section at the end of your paper that lists all the sources cited within the text. Here's how to structure and format the reference list:

1. Heading:

   - Center the title "References" at the top of the page.

   - Use the same font and font size as the rest of the paper (typically Times New Roman, 12-point).

2. Order of Entries:

   - List the entries in alphabetical order by the author's last name.

   - If a source has no author, use the title (or a shortened version) to alphabetize the entry.

3. Indentation:

   - Indent the second and subsequent lines of each entry (hanging indent).

   - The first line of each entry should be flush with the left margin, and subsequent lines should be indented by 0.5 inches.

4. Formatting:

- Use a consistent format for all entries, following the guidelines for each source type.

- Italicize the titles of books, journals, and other standalone works.

- Use sentence case for titles (capitalize only the first word, proper nouns, and the first word after a colon).

5. Punctuation:

- Use a period after each element of the reference entry (e.g., after the author's name, publication year, title, etc.).

- Use a comma to separate elements within the entry (e.g., between the author's name and publication year, between the title and publication year, etc.).

Formatting Guidelines for Different Source Types

In this section, we'll cover the specific formatting guidelines for various types of sources commonly cited in academic writing:

1. Books:

- Format: Author, A. A. (Year). Title of work. Publisher.

- Example: Smith, J. R. (2020). The Art of Academic Writing. Academic Press.

2. Journal Articles:

- Format: Author, A. A., Author, B. B., & Author, C. C. (Year). Title of article. Journal Title, volume(issue), page range.

- Example: Johnson, A., & Lee, K. (2019). Understanding student engagement. Journal of Educational Psychology, 25(3), 345-360.

3. Webpages:

   - Format: Author, A. A. (Year, Month Day). Title of webpage. Website Name. URL

   - Example: Smith, J. (2021, April 15). The Importance of Sleep. Sleep Foundation. https://www.sleepfoundation.org/importance-sleep-academic-success

4. Reports and Government Documents:

   - Format: Author, A. A. (Year). Title of report (Report No. xxx). Publisher.

   - Example: United Nations. (2020). Global Climate Change Report (Report No. 12345). United Nations Publications.

5. Other Source Types (e.g., conference proceedings, theses, personal communications):

   - Format varies depending on the type of source. Follow APA guidelines for each specific source type.

Handling Specific Citation Scenarios

In this section, we'll address how to handle specific citation scenarios when formatting entries in the reference list:

1. Citing Sources with No Author:

   - If a source has no author, begin the reference entry with the title of the work.

   - Use the first significant word of the title in place of the author's name when alphabetizing the entry.

   Example:

   - *Title of Article.* (2020). Journal Name, volume(issue), page range.

2. Citing Electronic Sources with No Date:

- If a source does not include a publication date, use "n.d." (no date) in place of the year in the reference entry.

- Provide as much detail as possible to help readers locate the source.

Example:

- Author, A. A. (n.d.). Title of Webpage. Website Name. Retrieved from URL

3. Citing Secondary Sources:

- When citing a source that you found cited in another source (a secondary source), list the original source in the reference list if possible.

- If you only have access to the secondary source, include both the original and secondary sources in the reference list.

Example:

- Original Source: Author, A. A. (Year). *Title of Original Work*. Publisher.
- Secondary Source: Author, B. B. (Year). *Title of Secondary Work*. Publisher.

4. Citing Translated Works:

- Include both the original publication year and the translation year in the reference entry.

- Place the original publication year in square brackets before the translator's name.

Example:

- Author, A. A. ([Original Year]). *Title of Work*. (Translator, Trans.).

CHAPTER 7: APPENDICES

In this chapter, we'll discuss the use of appendices in academic writing, particularly in APA style. Appendices are supplementary materials that provide additional information or data that is too lengthy or detailed to include in the main text of your paper. We'll cover the types of content that can be included in appendices, how to format them, and guidelines for referring to them within your paper.

Purpose and Content

Appendices serve the purpose of providing supplementary material that enhances the understanding of your paper's content without disrupting the flow of the main text. Here are some common types of content that can be included in appendices:

1. Raw Data: Appendices are often used to present raw data collected during research studies. This data may include survey responses, interview transcripts, or experimental results.

2. Additional Information: Appendices can contain additional information that supports the arguments or findings presented in the main text. This could include detailed descriptions of research methodologies, technical details, or mathematical derivations.

3. Visual Material: Tables, charts, graphs, and other visual aids that complement the main text can be included in appendices. These visuals help readers visualize complex information and provide supplementary context.

4. Documentation: Appendices can include supplementary documentation, such as consent forms, questionnaires, or interview protocols, that may be relevant to the research study but are not essential for understanding the main text.

5. Longer Textual Material: Occasionally, appendices may contain longer textual material, such as excerpts from documents, lengthy quotations, or translations, that are referenced in the main text but are too lengthy to include directly.

By including supplementary material in appendices, you can provide readers with access to additional information that enriches their understanding of your research without cluttering the main text.

Formatting and Organization

When formatting and organizing appendices in APA style, it's important to follow certain guidelines to ensure clarity and consistency. Here are some key points to consider:

1. Title and Labeling:

   - Each appendix should be clearly titled, using descriptive titles that indicate the content of the appendix (e.g., "Appendix A: Survey Questionnaire").

   - Appendices should be labeled alphabetically (e.g., Appendix A, Appendix B) if you have multiple appendices.

2. Placement:

   - Appendices should appear after the reference list and before any tables or figures in your paper.

   - Each appendix should begin on a new page.

3. Content Order:

   - Arrange the content of appendices in the order that it is mentioned in the main text of your paper.

   - Number or label tables, figures, or other visual material within each appendix sequentially (e.g., Table A1, Figure A1) to facilitate cross-referencing.

4. Formatting:

- Use the same font and font size as the rest of your paper for the content of appendices.

- If your paper has headings, use the same heading formatting (e.g., bold, italics) for headings in the appendices.

5. Referencing in the Text:

- In the main text of your paper, refer to appendices by their titles or labels (e.g., "see Appendix A for details").

- If you include specific information from an appendix, provide a clear citation to the relevant appendix in the text.

Following these formatting and organization guidelines will ensure that your appendices are well-structured and easy to navigate for readers.

Referring to and Citing Appendices

When referring to content from appendices within the main text of your paper, it's important to provide clear and concise references to guide readers to the relevant supplementary material. Here's how to refer to and cite appendices:

1. In-Text References:

- When referencing content from an appendix in the main text, provide a clear indication of where the reader can find the information.

- Use phrases such as "see Appendix A for details" or "refer to Appendix B for the full survey questionnaire" to direct readers to the relevant appendix.

2. Citations:

- If you directly cite or quote material from an appendix, include an in-text citation that corresponds to the relevant appendix.

- Use the title or label of the appendix (e.g., "Appendix A") in the in-text citation, followed by a brief description of the content being cited.

3. Placement of Citations:

- Place in-text citations to appendices immediately after the information being cited, within parentheses.

- If the citation refers to specific content within the appendix (e.g., a table or figure), provide additional details to help readers locate the information.

4. Consistency:

- Ensure consistency in how you refer to and cite appendices throughout your paper.

- Use the same format and style for referencing appendices in-text and in the reference list.

By providing clear references and citations to appendices, you help readers navigate your paper effectively and locate supplementary material that supports your arguments or findings.

CHAPTER 8: TABLES AND FIGURES

In this chapter, we'll discuss the use of tables and figures in academic writing, particularly in APA style. Tables and figures are visual representations of data or information that can enhance the presentation of your research findings. We'll cover the guidelines for creating and formatting tables and figures, as well as how to refer to them within your paper.

Purpose and Content

Tables and figures serve as visual aids to effectively present complex data or information in a clear and concise manner. They help readers understand key findings, trends, and relationships within your research. Here are some common types of content that can be presented using tables and figures:

1. Tables:

   - Tables are used to organize and present data in a structured format, making it easier to compare and analyze information.

   - They are often used to present numerical data, such as survey results, statistical analyses, or experimental findings.

   - Tables can also be used to summarize textual information or to provide detailed descriptions of research methodologies.

2. Figures:

   - Figures include various types of visual representations, such as graphs, charts, diagrams, maps, and photographs.

   - They are used to illustrate relationships, trends, patterns, or processes visually.

   - Figures are commonly used to present data that can be better understood visually, such as trends over time, distributions, or spatial relationships.

3. Combination of Text, Tables, and Figures:

   - Sometimes, a combination of text, tables, and figures may be used to present complex information comprehensively.

   - For example, a table may be accompanied by a figure to provide a visual summary of the data presented in the table, or vice versa.

By incorporating tables and figures into your paper, you can enhance the presentation of your research findings and facilitate readers' understanding of your work.

Creating and Formatting

When creating and formatting tables and figures in APA style, it's important to follow certain guidelines to ensure clarity, consistency, and accessibility. Here are some key points to consider:

1. Title and Numbering:

   - Each table and figure should be clearly titled to describe its content.

   - Tables and figures should be numbered sequentially (e.g., Table 1, Table 2, Figure 1, Figure 2) based on their order of appearance in the text.

2. Placement:

   - Place tables and figures as close as possible to the text where they are first mentioned.

   - If necessary, tables and figures can be placed on separate pages at the end of the paper following the reference list.

3. Formatting:

   - Use a consistent format for tables and figures throughout your paper, including font style, font size, and line spacing.

   - Ensure that text within tables and figures is legible and appropriately sized for readability.

4. Labeling:

- Tables should be labeled with the word "Table" followed by the table number and a brief descriptive title.

- Figures should be labeled with the word "Figure" followed by the figure number and a descriptive caption.

5. Notes and Sources:

- Provide any necessary notes or sources directly below the table or figure to explain abbreviations, define terms, or provide additional context.

- Use superscript lowercase letters (a, b, c) to indicate notes and sources, and provide corresponding explanations in a note section below the table or figure.

Following these guidelines will ensure that your tables and figures are well-formatted and effectively convey the information or data you wish to present.

Referring to Tables and Figures

When referring to tables and figures within the main text of your paper, it's important to provide clear and concise references to guide readers to the relevant visual aids. Here's how to refer to tables and figures:

1. In-Text References:

- When mentioning a table or figure in the text, provide a clear indication of its location and relevance to your discussion.

- Use phrases such as "as shown in Table 1" or "refer to Figure 2 for visual representation" to direct readers to the relevant visual aid.

2. Citations:

- If you directly cite or discuss information from a table or figure in the text, include a parenthetical citation to the corresponding table or figure.

- Use the table or figure number (e.g., Table 1, Figure 2) in the citation to indicate the source of the information.

3. Placement of References:

- Place references to tables and figures immediately after the information being cited, within parentheses.

- Ensure that references are placed close to the relevant discussion to maintain clarity and coherence.

4. Consistency:

- Maintain consistency in how you refer to tables and figures throughout your paper.

- Use the same format and style for referencing tables and figures in-text and in the reference list.

By providing clear references to tables and figures, you help readers navigate your paper effectively and locate visual aids that support your arguments or findings.

CHAPTER 9: CITATIONS OF ONLINE SOURCES

In this chapter, we'll discuss the specific considerations for citing online sources in APA style. With the increasing availability of digital information, it's essential to understand how to cite online sources accurately and effectively. We'll cover the formatting guidelines for various types of online sources, including websites, online articles, social media posts, and more. Additionally, we'll address how to handle URLs, DOIs, and retrieval dates in online citations.

Importance and General Principles

Accurately citing online sources is crucial for several reasons:

1. Scholarly Integrity: Citing sources appropriately acknowledges the work of others and upholds academic integrity by giving credit to the original authors.

2. Transparency: Providing citations allows readers to verify the information you've presented and locate the original sources for further exploration.

3. Avoiding Plagiarism: Proper citation practices help you avoid plagiarism by clearly distinguishing your ideas from those of others.

Here are some general principles to keep in mind when citing online sources:

1. Authorship: When possible, provide the author's name, whether it's an individual author, an organization, or a corporate entity.

2. Publication Date: Include the publication date of the online source to indicate its currency and relevance.

3. Title: Use the title of the webpage, article, or document as it appears on the site. Enclose the title in quotation marks if it's an article or webpage and italicize it if it's a standalone work.

4. URLs and DOIs: Include the URL (Uniform Resource Locator) or DOI (Digital Object Identifier) to provide readers with a direct link to the source. If a DOI is available, it's preferred over a URL as it provides a more stable link.

5. Retrieval Date: For online sources that may change over time (e.g., news articles, social media posts), include the date you accessed the source to indicate when you retrieved the information.

Adhering to these principles ensures that your citations are accurate, complete, and consistent with APA style guidelines.

Formatting Guidelines

When citing online sources in APA style, it's important to follow specific formatting guidelines to ensure accuracy and consistency. Here are the formatting guidelines for citing various types of online sources:

1. Websites:

  - Format: Author, A. A. (Year). Title of webpage. Website Name. URL

  - Example: Smith, J. (2022). How to cite online sources. Example.com. https://www.example.com/cite-online-sources

2. Online Articles:

  - Format: Author, A. A. (Year). Title of article. *Journal Name*, volume(issue), page range. DOI or URL

- Example: Johnson, K. (2021). The future of online education. *Journal of Educational Technology*, 10(2), 45-60. https://doi.org/10.1234/jet.2021.12345

3. Social Media Posts:

- Format: Author, A. A. [@username]. (Year, Month Day). Content of the post. Platform. URL

- Example: Davis, M. [@mdavis]. (2023, January 15). Excited to announce our new research project! #science #research. Twitter. https://twitter.com/mdavis/status/123456789

4. Online Videos:

- Format: Author, A. A. [Screen name]. (Year, Month Day). Title of video [Video]. Platform. URL

- Example: Smith, J. [ScienceExplorers]. (2022, May 1). Introduction to quantum mechanics [Video]. YouTube. https://www.youtube.com/watch?v=abcdef123456

5. Webpages with No Author:

- If no author is available, start the citation with the title of the webpage.

- Example: How to cite online sources. Example.com. https://www.example.com/cite-online-sources

Remember to include as much information as possible to help readers locate the online source. If a DOI is available, it's preferred over a URL. Additionally, include a retrieval date for sources that may change over time.

More Formatting Guidelines

6. E-books:

- Format: Author, A. A. (Year). *Title of Book*. Publisher. DOI or URL

- Example: Smith, J. (2020). *The Art of Academic Writing*. Academic Press. https://doi.org/10.1234/978-1-2345-6789-0

7. Online Reports and Whitepapers:

- Format: Author, A. A. (Year). *Title of Report* (Report No. xxx). Publisher. DOI or URL

- Example: Johnson, K. (2021). *State of Online Learning Report* (Report No. 123). Educational Research Institute. https://doi.org/10.1234/123456789

8. Online Forums and Discussion Boards:

- Format: Author, A. A. [Screen name]. (Year, Month Day). Title of post. Forum Name. URL

- Example: Miller, R. [rachelm]. (2023, February 10). Re: Online education trends. Education Forum. https://www.eduforum.com/topic/12345

9. Online Newspaper Articles:

- Format: Author, A. A. (Year, Month Day). Title of article. *Newspaper Name*. URL

- Example: Johnson, M. (2022, March 20). New study on online learning trends. *New York Times*. https://www.nytimes.com/2022/03/20/education/online-learning-study.html

10. Online Encyclopedia Entries:

- Format: Author, A. A. (Year). Title of entry. In *Title of Encyclopedia*. Publisher. URL

- Example: Smith, J. (2021). Online education. In *Encyclopedia of Education*. Encyclopedia Press. https://www.encyclopedia.com/education/online-education

When citing online sources, pay attention to details such as the author's name, publication date, title, and URL or DOI. Providing accurate and complete citations ensures that your readers can easily locate the sources you've referenced.

Additional Formatting Guidelines

11. Online Journals with No DOI:

   - Format: Author, A. A. (Year). Title of article. *Journal Name*, volume(issue), page range. URL

   - Example: Johnson, K. (2020). Trends in online education. *Journal of Educational Technology*, 8(3), 123-135. https://www.example.com/article123

12. Online Government Publications:

   - Format: Government Agency. (Year). *Title of Publication* (Publication No. xxx). Publisher. URL

   - Example: United States Department of Education. (2021). *National Education Report* (Publication No. 123). U.S. Government Printing Office. https://www.ed.gov/reports/national-education

13. Online Images:

   - Format: Creator, C. C. (Year). Title of image [Image]. Website Name. URL

   - Example: Smith, J. (2022). Online education infographic [Image]. Educational Trends. https://www.edutrends.com/online-education-infographic

14. Online Podcasts:

   - Format: Host, H. H. (Year, Month Day). Title of episode [Audio podcast episode]. Podcast Name. URL

   - Example: Johnson, K. (2023, April 5). Online learning strategies [Audio podcast episode]. Education Talks. https://www.edutalks.com/online-learning-strategies

15. Online Interviews:

   - Format: Interviewee, I. I. (Year, Month Day). Title of interview. Interviewed by Interviewer Name [Format]. Publisher. URL

- Example: Smith, J. (2022, May 10). Future of online education. Interviewed by K. Johnson [Interview]. Educational Insights. https://www.edinsights.com/online-education-interview

Following these guidelines will help ensure that your citations of online sources are accurate, consistent, and compliant with APA style.

Handling URLs, DOIs, and Retrieval Dates

When citing online sources in APA style, it's important to include relevant information such as URLs, DOIs, and retrieval dates to help readers locate the sources. Here's how to handle these elements in online citations:

1. URLs (Uniform Resource Locators):

   - Include the full URL of the webpage or online source in the citation.

   - Ensure that the URL is accurate and functional, allowing readers to access the source directly.

   - Do not use "https://" or "http://" in the URL unless required by the publisher or if the URL begins with "www."

2. DOIs (Digital Object Identifiers):

   - Include the DOI if available for the online source. DOIs provide a permanent link to the source and are preferred over URLs.

   - If a DOI is provided, use it instead of the URL in the citation.

   - Format DOIs as URLs by adding "https://doi.org/" before the DOI number.

3. Retrieval Dates:

   - Include a retrieval date for online sources that may change over time, such as news articles or social media posts.

- Use the format "Retrieved Month Day, Year" (e.g., Retrieved May 1, 2024) followed by a period.

Here's an example of a citation with a URL, DOI, and retrieval date:

- Author, A. A. (Year). Title of webpage. Website Name. https://www.example.com/cite-online-sources. doi:10.1234/123456789. Retrieved May 1, 2024.

Including URLs, DOIs, and retrieval dates in online citations ensures that your readers have the necessary information to access and verify the sources you've referenced.

Summary

In this chapter, we discussed the specific considerations for citing online sources in APA style. Here's a summary of the key points covered:

1. Importance of Accurate Citations: Accurately citing online sources is essential for scholarly integrity, transparency, and avoiding plagiarism.

2. General Principles: When citing online sources, include the author's name, publication date, title, URL or DOI, and retrieval date (if necessary).

3. Formatting Guidelines: Follow specific formatting guidelines for different types of online sources, including websites, online articles, social media posts, and more.

4. Handling URLs, DOIs, and Retrieval Dates: Include the full URL of the source, use DOIs when available, and include retrieval dates for sources that may change over time.

5. Consistency and Clarity: Maintain consistency in formatting and citation style throughout your paper, and ensure that citations are clear and easy to follow for readers.

By adhering to these guidelines, you can effectively cite online sources in your academic writing, ensuring accuracy, transparency, and compliance with APA style.

CHAPTER 10: CONCLUSION AND FURTHER RESOURCES

In this final chapter, we'll conclude our guide to APA style and provide additional resources for further exploration. We'll summarize the key points covered in this guide and offer suggestions for where to find more information on APA style, including online resources, books, and academic journals.

Summarizing the key points covered in this guide to APA style:

Summary

In this guide to APA style, we covered various aspects of academic writing following the guidelines of the 7th edition of the APA Manual. Here's a summary of the key points covered:

1. Title Page and Formatting: We discussed the elements of the title page, including the title, author name, and institutional affiliation, and provided guidelines for formatting.

2. In-Text Citations: We explained how to format and punctuate in-text citations, including author-date citations and direct quotations, as well as how to handle specific citation scenarios.

3. Reference List: We outlined the structure and formatting guidelines for creating a reference list, including the order of entries, indentation, and formatting rules for different source types.

4. Appendices: We discussed the purpose and content of appendices, as well as guidelines for formatting and organizing appendices in your paper.

5. Tables and Figures: We covered the guidelines for creating, formatting, and referring to tables and figures within your paper.

6. Citations of Online Sources: We provided specific formatting guidelines for citing various types of online sources, including websites, online articles, social media posts, and more, and discussed how to handle URLs, DOIs, and retrieval dates.

Overall, following the guidelines outlined in this guide will help you maintain consistency, accuracy, and clarity in your academic writing in accordance with APA style.

Further Resources

1. APA Manual: The Publication Manual of the American Psychological Association (7th edition) is the authoritative source for APA style guidelines. It provides comprehensive guidance on all aspects of academic writing, citation, and formatting.

2. APA Style Website: The official APA Style website (https://apastyle.apa.org/) offers a wealth of resources, including tutorials, FAQs, blog posts, and sample papers, to help you navigate APA style.

3. APA Style Blog: The APA Style Blog (https://apastyle.apa.org/blog) is a valuable resource for answering specific questions about APA style, clarifying common issues, and staying updated on the latest developments in APA style guidelines.

4. APA Journals: Many journals published by the American Psychological Association follow APA style guidelines for manuscript submission and formatting. Consulting articles published in APA journals can provide examples of APA style in practice.

5. Books on APA Style: There are several books available that provide detailed guidance on APA style, including "Publication Manual of the American Psychological Association" (7th edition), "APA Style Simplified" by Bernard C. Beins, and "APA Made Easy" by Scott Matkovich.

6. Online Writing Centers: Many universities and colleges offer online writing centers with resources and tutorials on academic writing, including APA style. Check if your institution provides access to such resources.

By utilizing these further resources, you can deepen your understanding of APA style and enhance your proficiency in academic writing.

This concludes our guide to APA style. We hope you found it helpful, and we wish you success in your academic endeavors!

Made in the USA
Middletown, DE
22 August 2024

59588090R00038